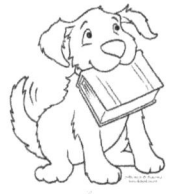

Beyond Fertility
Crossing the Bridge of Life

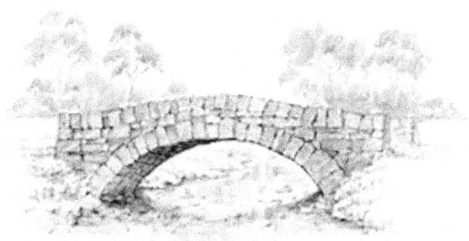

K. B. LeMere, ND

Health by Design Publishing
Dallas, Texas

I am blessed to have three loving men in my life:

my husband for the hours of time together he has given up,

my son for his encouragement to press on,

my father who taught me I can do anything through Christ that strengths me .

This book is dedicated to them.

Beyond Fertility
Crossing the Bridge of Life

Copyright © 2016

By K.B. LeMere, ND

E-book

Health by Design Publishing

Author Information

Email: drklemere@gmail.com

Web: www.author-kblemere.com

Book in Print

ISBN 9781543208443

9 781543 208443

Printed in the United States of America

Contents

Section 1 Introduction

Section 2 Stages

Section 3. Medical Views

Section 4. Symptoms

Section 5. Hormone Replacement Therapy

Section 6. Beyond Fertility

Section 7. Going Natural, Herbal ,Formulas and Tips

Section 8. Nutrition

Section 9. Men

Section 10. Couples

Introduction

The train is coming down the track at full speed how do I get off? The age is 50 for both men and women. Your body is at the controls; the closer the train gets to the bridge the slower and slower it gets in order to prepare for the crossing. Stacey Coling, a writer for More magazines, describes it like puberty in reverse; your body is riding a hormonal roller coaster.

For the men and women in there fifties, like young people in their teens, everything seems to change. Women's ovaries are gearing down for the retirement called menopause. Your children start beating you at games, print grows smaller, rooms lack enough light to read, and your skin loses its elasticity. The body takes on wrinkles, bulges and begins to sag. Men lose hair they want to keep;

women grow hair they want to lose. Does not sound pretty!

Technically, menopause arrives one year after your final period. You may find yourself gazing back into the past and analyzing what your accomplishments you have made therefore, thinking about where we are going. At about age 60 to 65, we begin living for the first time in our lives between sunrise and sunset. Most people stop marching forward from birthday to birthday, numbering their years, but instead they look at how many years they have left. In these middle years, it forces us to take stock of ourselves. A man who has been trying to reach the top realizes he will never get there. He must settle for some place in between. In addition, a man, who has reached the top, looks back and wonders if it was worth the time and sacrifices.

The medical profession is not exactly leading the way for women in menopause. Instead, women are turning to alternative methods and reclaiming their bodies and health by taking back their power and their lives.

Once your body settles down and accepts the change, you are finally on the other side of menopause (post). You have crossed the bridge. You will have a glow, an energy that is magnetic, you will be full of integrity, joy, overflowing with love and have a sense of self-pride and worth. The midlife opens up promises and possibilities if we seize it as a teachable moment in life. Keep a positive perspective concerning potential and accept new challenges.

What have your accomplishments been, to date?
Where are you going from here?
What have you learned?
What knowledge, talents, and abilities can you take forward
to the other side of the bride?

Stages

Am I Loosing My Mind?

Menopause is divided into three phases. Phase 1 is prior to menopause or premenopausal, during this time women usually ovulate irregularly due to either inadequate secretion of estrogen or resistance of the remaining follicles to ovulatory stimulus. Phase 2 is often called perimenopause or the menopausal transition. It can last anywhere from four years to ten and is unnervingly unpredictable. Some women have normal periods all the way through this phase until the last one ends. Other women have periods that come a week early or a week late, then skip an entire month. Margery Gass, MD, executive director of the North American Menopause Society and a consultant at the Cleveland Clinic Center for Specialized Women's Health says,"It's normal to reach menopause between the ages of 41 and 55, with 51 being the average." Smokers tend to experience menopause a year sooner than other women. During phase 3 your body accepts the change, you have crossed the bridge. The other side, midlife, opens up promises and possibilities for new challenges.

The three phases have no particular time periods. Each women experiences them differently in terms of when each phase starts, how long it lasts and what kind of symptoms appear. Symptoms such as hot flashes, tender breasts, insomnia and headaches are a normal part of menopause. Nancy Santoro, MD, chair of obstetrics and gynecology at the University of Colorado School of Medicine in Denver says, "some women are just much more sensitive to the hormonal changes than others".

The International Panel of Women's Health experts have established a criteria called the STRAW +10 Staging System. STRAW stands for Stages of Reproductive Aging Workshop.

STRAW + 10 Staging System

Stage 1 Late Reproductive Years

Transition before perimenopause - This is the final stage of the baby-making years, a time when your ability to have a child declines rapidly. This stage can continues up to 9 years.

Stage 2 Early Menopausal Transition

This is the beginning of perimenopause, This usually last 4 or more years.

Stage 3 Late Menopausal Transition

The second full-fledged phase of perimenopause often occurs at about age 49. This is the highest time to be affected by symptoms. This stage last generally one to three years.

Stage 4 Easy Post-menopause

At this stage, you've recently crossed to the other side of menopause; in other words, you've gone more than a year without a period. First part: 2 years. Remaining part: 3 to 6 years.

Symptoms are thought to occur when there are no longer any eggs left in the ovaries. At birth, there are about one million eggs; at puberty, the number drops to about 400,000 and only 400 of these eggs actually mature during reproductive years. By the time a woman reaches fifty, few eggs remain. The absence of the cellular housing of the egg results in reduced production of estrogen and progesterone. The body responds to the reduced estrogen by the pituitary gland increasing secretion of follicle-stimulating hormone (FSH) and luteinizing hormone (LH). This also happens with surgical menopause brought on by a full hysterectomy.

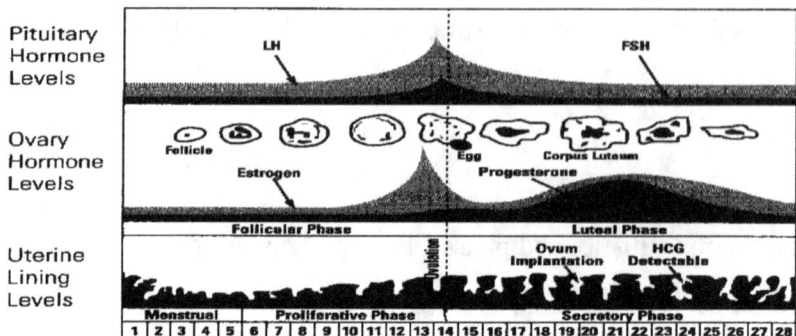

The period after menopause is referred to as postmenopausal. But, what causes it? After menopause, FSH and LH are secreted in large and continuous quantities. LH and FSH cause the ovaries and the adrenal glands to secrete increased amounts of androgens, which can be converted to estrogens by the fat cells of the hips and thighs. Converted androgens account for most of the circulating estrogen in the postmenopausal woman, but the total estrogen levels are still far below the levels for reproductive function. Most medical professionals are not exactly leading the way for women in menopause; instead, women are turning to alternative methods and reclaiming their bodies and health by taking back their power and lives.

Medical Views

Today, women are steadily confronted with a stream of advertisements about hormones, making them feel it is a natural step to take when menopause begins. These decisions are not to be taken lightly. No one tells us we have choices. When a woman today goes to her doctors, she is seeking advise and education on the subject of estrogen replacement and menopause. The physicians look at menopause as a disease in need of treatment, thus prescribing estrogen. Traditional medical doctors are trained to listen to symptoms and give you something to eliminate those symptoms thus, prescribing estrogen. The current medical treatment of menopause primarily involves the use of hormone replacement therapy, HRT, utilizing a combination of estrogen and progesterone. Medical doctors use primarily two criteria's in diagnosing menopause:

1. The cessation of menstruation between the ages of 40 and 55
2. Going six to twelve months without a period

If you don't fall into one of these categories, your symptoms are considered PMS related. I say most doctors because if you are lucky enough to find a doctor that will listen to your symptoms and work with you using natural therapies, you have found a special gift. Hold on to them.

Naturopathic doctors listen to the symptoms but they are like detectives, they look for the root cause of the symptoms and try to work with you using natural remedies.

The advertising public and the allopathic doctors send the message that unless menopause is medically managed, women will end up dry, brittle, parched, and devoid of life. The ads proclaim that aging is to be feared, that it is impossible to remain strong or attractive without the benefit of taking estrogen. More than 5 million women take estrogens. Nevertheless, do they know what the side effects are? The Physicians' Desk Reference provides a long list of side effects of HRT, as do the package inserts for estrogen and progesterone products.

This is what the patient information sheet says on the hormone patch:

Warning-Dangers of Estrogens

Cancer of the uterus The risk of developing cancer of the uterus gets higher the longer estrogens are used and when larger doses are taken.

Cancer of the breast Studies that examine the risk of breast cancer among women using estrogen along with combined estrogen/progestin therapy, suggest that there may be mildly increased risk of breast cancer in women taking the combined therapy.

Gallbladder disease Women who use estrogens after menopause are more likely to develop gallbladder disease, needing surgery, than women who do not use estrogens.

Abnormal blood clotting Taking estrogens may increase the risk of blood clots. These clots can cause a stroke, heart attack, or pulmonary embolus, any of which may be fatal.

These drugs have been implicated in the causation of gall bladder disease and cancer of the uterus. In spite of the FDA warnings to doctors and patients, they are still being prescribed and taken. Estrogen therapy is said to preserve youth, relieve depression, prevent cardiovascular disease and to prevent bone demineralization. Other side effects listed are nausea, breast tenderness, depression, liver disorders, adult-onset asthma and enlargement of uterine fibroids, fluid retention, blood sugar disturbances, and headaches.

Exercise and diet can also prevent demineralization. My hope is that you will gain knowledge from this book and be able to make a determination of what is best for you.

Symptoms

There are several symptoms all women share with difference of severity. These symptoms are due to the rapid decrease in estrogen levels. They are: night sweats, hot flashes, osteoporosis, heart disease, mood swings, headaches, atrophic vaginitis, bladder infections, cold hands and feet, forgetfulness and inability to concentrate. It is not unusual to have all these symptoms.

Many of these symptoms, particularly hot flashes, are a result of altered function of the hypothalamus, which is a mass of nervous tissue at the center of the brain that serves as the bridge between the nervous systems and the hormonal endocrine system. The hypothalamus is responsible for the control of many body functions, body temperature, metabolic rate, sleep patterns, reactions to stress, libido, mood and the release of pituitary hormones. The bodies own mood elevating and pain-relieving compounds are the functioning of the hypothalamus when endorphins are released. Endorphins are thought to play a role in hot flashes. Some of the beneficial effects against hot flashes could be from enhancing endorphin output. This can be obtained this through exercise and acupuncture. A study has been done on each of these with interesting facts to help women understand why they are having these symptoms and what they can do about them. An estimated 75 percent of women experience hot flashes during the transition. Night sweats that occur while sleeping are also very common; these two discomforts are classified as vasomotor symptoms. Obese women are more likely to get hot flashes because the fat tissue makes their bodies warmer.

Hot Flashes and Night Sweats: They are episodes of intense heat and sweating. They are a dilation of the peripheral blood vessels, which leads to a rise in skin temperature and flushing of the skin. During a hot flash, the skin, especially the head and neck, become red and warm for a few seconds to two minutes, with cold chills after. They can be accompanied by other symptoms like increased heart rate, headaches, dizziness, weight gain, fatigue, and insomnia. The insomnia is usually because at night, a woman may soak her sheets with perspiration.

Slow, deep breathing can make them feel less intense. The breathing will help dial down your physiological reaction. A 2005 study found that women who practiced slow deep breathing experienced almost 50 percent fewer episodes. As you breathe, keep your rib cage still, lower, and raise your diaphragm to fill and empty your lungs. Inhale for five seconds, pushing your stomach muscles out, then exhale for five seconds, pulling your stomach muscles in and up.

These hot flashes are not usually visible to others. Estrogen is effective in reducing or elimination hot flashes, however estrogen only postpones the symptoms, when estrogen is stopped they return. There are other proven methods to deal with hot flashes. Women who do aerobic exercise regularly and eat healthy vegetarian diets, have less frequent and severe hot flashes.

Women who take 200 mg of vitamin C along with 200 mg of bioflavonoids six times a day received complete relief. In a recent Turkish study, the severity of hot flashes declined in women who received acupuncture twice a week. Another study at the Ankara Training and Research Hospital did find heightened levels of estrogen in women who underwent a series of acupuncture sessions along with taking traditional Chinese herbs.

Vitamin E supplements, hypnosis, yoga, meditation, homeopathic remedies, ginseng, and other herbs including black cohosh and Chase berry tea have all been clinically effective. Two herbal capsules three times a day of equal parts licorice root, burdock root, wild yam root, dong quay root and motherwort have proven to remove hot flashes. Hot flashes are the worst during the first two years. After the body adapts to decreased estrogen levels, hot flashes subside.

Aromatherapy Tip:

Carry the essential oil of *Clergy Sage*. Putting some on a handkerchief and smelling it, will immediate relieve symptoms of a hot flash or night sweats!

Headaches: Menopause headaches are due to increased instability of the blood vessels. Menstrual migraines are due to the rise and fall of estrogen levels and can cause headaches to become more frequent. Identify triggers such as alcohol, certain foods, weather changes, stress or anything else that brings it on.

Irregular Periods: If you are having irregular periods, first rule out any possibility pregnancy. If you miss two periods in a row, take an over the counter pregnancy test. Make an appointment with your doctor. Consider taking low-dose contraceptives if erratic bleeding patterns are driving you crazy. Doctors will typically steer you away from taking oral contraceptives if you have a history of blood clots, heart disease, breast cancer or endometrial cancer or if you smoke. A gynecologist will have multiple prescribed solutions.

Mood Changes: Do you have edginess or irritability? It is a common PMS perimenopause symptom. Vitamin D is linked to improved mood; New research from the University of Minnesota found that women who consumed less than 400 IU of vitamin D daily had significantly lower scores on mental-health quality-of-life measures, than those who consumed more than 400 IU per day.

Breast Tenderness: If your breast feel swollen and achy, it could be because you're not ovulating regularly, says Jan Shifren, MD, director of the Vincent Menopause Program at Massachusetts General Hospital in Boston. Cold packs can provide relief.

Forgetfulness: You walk into a room and forget what it was you came for, you have trouble paying attention or focusing on what you're supposed to be doing. This brain fog is due to hormonal changes, sleep disturbances, depression, or stress overload. Here is some good news: caffeine gives you a mental boost, so have that cup or two of coffee in the morning. In a study of women ages 40 to 60, who complained of memory loss, results showed problems on "working memory," which is the ability to hold data. An example would be, looking at your restaurant bill and not being able to calculate the tip. A possible solution is talking to your doctor about a non stimulant drug used for AD. These are common symptoms due to the age of the women in menopause or a decreased oxygen and nutrient supply to the brain. In older women, it could be atherosclerosis, hardening of the arteries, of the blood vessels supplying oxygen and nutrition to the brain. The brain is highly dependent on a constant supply of oxygen and nutrients. It weighs only 3 pounds; the brain utilizes about twenty percent of the oxygen supply of the entire body. The goal is to feed the brain with a supply of blood, oxygen and nutrients. I recommend adding liquid oxygen to your water. Products like Oxy Up and Oxygen drops can be purchased online from a company called Inner light.

Insomnia: According to sleep experts, 40 percent of menopausal women experience disrupted sleep. For more information, click on "The Stress Reduction Program" at the site of the Center for Mindfulness in Medicine, Health Care and Society at the University of Massachusetts Medical School. Try taking Benadryl, it will help you fall asleep and is safe.

Osteoporosis: Bone is living tissue. New bone is constantly being made, and old bone is constantly being taken up or reabsorbed. The two processes should be in balance, but if more bone is lost than made, the bones become brittle and can break easily. ERT is widely used to slow bone re-absorption in menopausal women. Advertisements would like us to believe that the hormones Premarin or Estradiol are the answer to everything as they imply they prevent bones from dissolving. Important: What they don't tell you is when you take ERT there is no different time as to how long you must take it and if you choose to stop after four years the rate of bone loss can increase greatly. So, please realize, once you decide to take hormones, it is best to stay on them. I am speaking from experience. In 1992, I had a hysterectomy due to Endometriosis. While in the hospital the doctor immediate started me on Estrogen. After understanding what I do now, several years ago I tried to go natural. The pain I suffered in my bones was unbelievable. I suffered for three months. I just got stiffer and stiffer until I could hardly function, so I went back on the estrogen patch. Within 72 hours, I was pain free and mobile.

Statistics support the fact that osteoporosis is only a problem for meat and dairy eaters. Females meat-eaters at the age of 65 have lost 35 percent of their bone mass and female vegetarians at the same age only have a loss of 18 percent. Dairy products are not the best source of calcium because the calcium they contain is from animal protein. The best sources of calcium are from green leafy vegetables, tofu, broccoli and sunflower seeds.

Exercise is very important to keep bone mass increasing. Women who have a healthy lifestyle have far less bone mass loss than those women that smoke, drink alcohol, caffeine, cola drinks and eat salt and sugar. Women who do not want to take prescription drugs should try these alternative methods: eat a vegetarian diet without dairy; exercise daily by walking 30 minutes a day and use natural wild yam cream applied to the skin 4 times a day.

Heart Disease The medical profession has proven that estrogen taken for long periods does lower rates of heart disease and cholesterol. However, women who eat a low-fat, high-fiber vegetarian-type diet obtain these same benefits without drugs. You do have choices, but diet control is not easy.

Cold Hands and Feet: There are three major causes of cold hands and feet related to menopause: hypothyroidism, low iron levels in the body, and poor circulation. Appropriate blood testing must be obtained to determine which of the three needs treatment. If it is Hypothyroid you will notice dry skin, hair falling out, brain fog and several other dominate symptoms.

Atrophic Vaginitis or vaginal dryness: The cause of this is due to hormone levels dropping. The vaginal lining becomes thinner, drier, and less elastic due to lack of estrogen. As a result, the vagina becomes sore and irritated by sexual intercourse, increased susceptibility to infections, and symptoms of vaginal itching or burning. Usually estrogen cream is prescribed for this. The alternative answer is using lubricants such as castor oil, vitamin E or soluble jellies and natural progesterone cream.

Bladder Infections: About 15% of menopausal women experience frequent bladder infections. During menopause, there is a breakdown in natural defense mechanisms that protect against bacterial growth in the urinary tract. An example would be to enhance the flow of urine by achieving and maintaining proper hydration, promoting a pH that will inhibit the growth of the organism, and preventing bacterial adherence to the endothelial cells of the bladder. To measure your pH, check first morning urine and saliva. Check the color against the color chart that comes in the kit. Nature Sunshine has several herbs for bladder problems, the combination KA or URY are two of them. I think the best herbs are from a company called (www.Rain-tree.com). Order Urinary Support.

Tips:

1. Use vitamin E 1000 IU gel cap inserted into the vagina at night before bed.

2. Women should try to avoid substances that tend to dry the mucous membranes, including antihistamines, alcohol, caffeine, and diuretics. It is critical that the body stay well hydrated. Drinking at least 64 ounces of water daily is imperative. As a nutritionist, I bug my clients about this. If you don't listen to anything I say, at least drink 64 ounces of pure water. Why? The body is 80% water. Your body will naturally lose at least 64 ounces of water a day through urine, sweat, fecal elimination, and other sources. When you don't put back the water your body needs, it becomes more and more dehydrated until you become ill.

3. Underwear and clothes made from natural fibers such as cotton are best because they allow the skin to breathe, thus decreasing the incidence of vaginal infections. Regular intercourse is a benefit, as it increases blood flow to vaginal tissues, which helps improve tone and lubrications.

4. Mood swings and depression studies showed women taking estrogen for depression and mood swings became less outwardly aggressive but more inwardly hostile. Following the above alternative methods will alleviate these symptoms. Try an herbal supplement such as Sam-E.

Hormone Replacement Therapy

HRT Facts

Women are steadily confronted with a stream of advertisements about hormones, making them feel it is a natural step to begin taking ERT (estrogen replacement therapy) at menopause. The ads proclaim that it is impossible to remain strong and attractive without the benefit of estrogens. More than 5 million women take estrogens. However, do they ask about the side effects? The Physicians' Desk Reference provides a long list of side effects of HRT, as do the package inserts as previously described.

Hormone therapy is typically a combination of estrogen and progesterone for women who've had hysterectomies. Estrogen alone is the quickest and easiest way to alleviate the symptoms. JoAnn Manson, MD a professor of medicine at Harvard Medical School, developed a flowchart that takes risks and benefits into account. The key factor is whether menopausal symptoms are impairing your quality of life, in which case you might consider hormone therapy. Below are the questions on her flow chart.

1. *Do you have significant symptoms of menopause – moderate to severe hot flashes or night sweats? Answer No - HT isn't recommended; Answer Yes - read on.*

2. *Do you have a history of heart disease, stroke, transient ischemic attack (mini stroke) or breast cancer? Answer No - read on; Answer Yes - HT isn't recommended*

3. *Have you ever had a blood cot in your leg or deep vein thrombosis? Answer Yes - transdermal estrogen may be an option; Answer No - read on*

4. *How many years has it been since your last menstrual period? 5 or less, read on; 6 to 10 read on; more than 10, HT not right for you.*

If it's been five years or less since your last period and your risk of heart disease over the next 10 years is: very low less than 5%: HT is ok; moderate 10-20%: Transdermal HT is ok; high more than 20%: no HT.

If it's been six to 10 years since your last period and your risk of heart disease over the next 10 years is: very low, less than 5%: HT is ok; low 5-10% or moderate: transdermal HT is ok; high more than

20%: No HT

In my research, it was interesting to see the history of estrogen replacement therapy in society. The chart below shows the progression in years.

History of ERT (Estrogen Replacement Therapy)

- **1938** - Synthetic estrogen was discovered by Dr. Charles Dood

- **1960** - A gynecologist Robert Wilson, M.D., concluded that menopausal women needed ERT to prevent death of their womanhood. His research was financed by Wyeth-Ayerst

- **1966** - Robert Wilson published the book "Feminine Forever" saying that ERT would rescue women from old age

- **1975** - Six million women, one third of those over 50 were taking estrogen replacement drugs manufactured by Wyeth-Ayerst

- **1988** - Ciba-Geigy began sponsoring educational seminars around the country led by local doctors about ERT using the Estradiol patch

- **1992** - Wyeth-Ayerst spent $9 million advertising Premarin in women's magazines alone and Ciba-Geigy spent $5 million on ads for the Estradiol patch

- **1993** - Gallup survey showed 84% of American physicians discussed with their patients about menopausal symptoms centered on ERT. Fewer than 2% discussed natural approaches

- **1994** - Time magazine featured a cover story acknowledging the drawbacks to taking estrogen

- **2001** - 95% of Physicians still do not take the time to educate their patients about choice or natural therapies

- **2002** – WHI study stopped the combined estrogen and progesterone HRT arm of the study prematurely in light of findings of safety issues, which combined HRT – a small increased risk of breast cancer, heart disease, stroke and blood clots

- **2003** - Both doctors and HRT users are confused regarding safety issues. Many doctors advise their patients to come off HRT. Such actions were, and continue to be, unduly influenced by a high level of media interest that has tended to attract some health scare headlines.

- **2004** – HRT users fall from 2 million to less than 1 million in the UK

- **2007** – Show previous studies results were over-estimated. These show additional benefits of HRT use for those 50-59 age group.

- **2012** - Publication of a Danish study of combined HRT use for 10 years in healthy women started shortly after menopause showing reduced heart disease and mortality.

- **2017** - The beliefs remain the same, that HRT reduces heart disease and bone demineralization.

As I stated earlier, HRT drugs are implicated to be the causation of gall bladder disease and cancer of the uterus, but in spite of the FDA warnings to doctors and patients, they are still prescribing them for our comfort. Why? Estrogen therapy is said to preserve youth, relieve depression, and prevent cardiovascular disease. So, when women are told this, who wouldn't want to take ERT just to preserve their youth! Guess what, exercise and diet can also prevent demineralization. It is not as easy as taking a pill but a lot healthier.

There are many types of replacement therapy, so how do we know which one is the best? Women that choose to use hormone replacement therapy may do so for a short-term period or may need to do so if they have a very high risk for osteoporosis. If you choose to take HRT, consider the following:

A combined continuous hormone replacement therapy is the best in terms of benefit-to-risk ratio. Try natural estrogen first; like Conjugated estrogens (Premarin, Genesis), Esterified estrogen (Evex, Menest), Micronized 17-beta estradiol (Estrace), Transdermal 17-beta estradiol (Estradiol, System) and TripleEstrogen (Tri-Est).

There are other types of HRT. When estrogen is given without progestin, it is known as unopposed estrogen therapy. The most commonly used forms are mixtures of excreted estrogens obtained from mare's urine, called conjugated estrogen. Conjugated estrogens are metabolized in the body into active forms of estrogen, such as 17-beta-estradiol. Unfortunately, the liver breaks down many of the active estrogens before they have the opportunity to produce their effects. Therefore, large amounts of conjugated estrogens are given because they are not well absorbed orally, but they are absorbed well through the skin using estrogen patches and vaginal creams. Patches are preferable because they deliver estrogens within the female body's natural secretions into the bloodstream in a slow manner.

Natural physicians use triple estrogen or Tri-Est. This is a combination of three major natural forms of estrogen: estriol, estrone, and estradiol.

In most cases, hormone replacement therapy is not necessary. Symptoms can be managed using natural therapies. Keep in mind each of us have different severities of symptoms. Some women suffer such severe symptoms they become suicidal. Menopause can feel like a "thorn in your side" or "your cross to bear". A thorn in your side was Paul's example of a disability that he must rely on Christ to overcome. A cross to bear is a weight or burden you carry and must rely on the Lord to help you.

For women at high risk of osteoporosis and women who have already experienced significant bone loss, hormone replacement therapy may be appropriate. For me it was not a choice. My mother and her mother both had Osteo and Rheumatoid Arthritis. I began with signs and symptoms in my late 20's ending in a hysterectomy at 44.

The natural approach to counteract the symptoms of menopause is to focus on improving physiology. This can be done through diet, nutritional supplementation, the use of herbs, and exercise. The nutrients, which are proven effective in relieving hot flashes and atrophic vaginitis in clinical studies are vitamin E, vitamin C, and Ferulic acid (an abundant phenolic phytochemical found in plant cell wall components) along with dietary recommendations and an exercise program.

The only clinical studies done on vitamin E were in late 1940s. They found vitamin E to be effective in relieving hot flashes and menopausal vaginal complaints plus improve the blood supply to the vaginal wall when taken for at least four weeks. In 1949, a follow-up study was published stating 400 IU of vitamin E was effective in treating atrophic vaginitis. Vitamin E oil, creams, ointments, or suppositories can be used topically to provide relief of atrophic vaginitis. Vitamin E suggested dosage is 800 IU per day until symptoms have improved, then 400 IU per day. I suggest inserting the vitamin E vaginally as described earlier.

Beyond Fertility

Encouragement

Menopause - the cessation of a woman's monthly periods - announces the retirement of her ovaries from active duty and thus the end of her childbearing years. Aging and physical changes occurring after menopause are considered a negative because there can be unpleasant physical repercussions. Yet, there is a season of time for all things. Let me encourage you to honor the wisdom that comes with aging.

I believe God made clear that there is a season for all things (Ecc. 3:1-12) Events take place on heaven's timeline, but God encourages us to focus on today, to honor the wisdom that comes with aging (Job 12:12) and to serve Him in our own lifetime by doing good (Ecc. 3:12)

Take a minute to pause and make a list. Come up with three post-menopausal women that stand out as key figures to you. Someone who thought herself too old to be of any use but yet was an essential contributor to your rearing. Mine was my grandmother who always had something positive and encouraging to say. Next, think of two women you consider wise and godly, who were instrumental in your lineage or life events.

My inspiration comes from the bible: Three post-menopausal women stand out as key figures in the bible, Naomi, who thought herself too old to be of any use in Ruth's life (Ruth 1:12), was essential in the courtship of Ruth and Boaz and contributed to the rearing of their son Obed (Ruth 4:16-17). Both Sarah and Elizabeth in their old age conceived and bore sons who played important roles in the kingdom (Gen. 18:11; Luke 1:36). Each of these wise and godly women were instrumental in the familial lineage or events surrounding the birth of Jesus Christ.

Enjoyment of post-menopausal years in healthy activity is often a matter of personal choice and planning. The uncomfortable physical symptoms of menopause can be avoided or minimized by working with a physician, nutritionist, naturopath, or herbalist. You are valuable and your age has nothing to do with the knowledge and experience you can offer to others.

At some time, all women and men have passed over the bridge into a new season of life called menopause. Men's bodies decrease in testosterone and women's bodies decrease in estrogen. Each of us are made of different personality types therefore we each deal with these life changes in different ways. Our bodies are in preparation to stop producing children.

Until the late 1980s, families were in the "Leave It to Beaver" mode. Most women devoted their lives to raising their children, being a helpmate to their husbands, keeping their home and giving to their church and community. In the 1990s came a different concept. Women took full time positions, focused on higher education, and new laws were passed for divorce called irreconcilable differences, which in turn forced families to come second and produced latch key kids. This driving and pushing through life forces families to go in different direction, but then something happens between the ages of 40 and 50. After we cross the bridge, a new season of thinking begins to take place. We begin to slow down and not only look back as to where we have been and what we have accomplished but also look ahead as to what we want to do with the rest of our lives. Where are we going? This change usually beings when the last child graduates from high school and prepares to leave home.

After the children are gone some women's thoughts begin to flourish implying it's their turn in life to do whatever they want. It's a feeling of celebration. I home schooled our youngest son all the way through high school. It was a delightful time for us as a family. We used the opportunity to travel and experience the things we were studying. For his senior year, he was ready for college, so he took the SAT's and scored so high that Dallas Baptist University admitted him as a Freshman in college, plus giving him credit for his senior year of high school. I sold my business and came up with a new life plan.

What do you do with forty plus years of wisdom, and knowledge? As older women, we are to educating the younger women into knowledge. At 46, I did not feel like the older woman, I felt young, healthy, and wanted to do something meaningful. First I had to take care of the endometriosis that had been causing me so much pain. It was time for that hysterectomy.

After a woman's fertile years are over she has a purpose and that is not to wither away and die. Just because we have outlived our ovaries, we have not outlived our usefulness. This is our time to enjoy life trying those things we have always wanted to do and have dreamed about, but didn't take the time to do. Some women go back to school to finish a degree and some find a career.

For some women it is a time of depression. They wake up one day and realize they have devoted their entire lives to nurturing and building a relationship with their children and their young adult children are now leaving with joy to start their new life. These women don't know what they are going to do with the rest of their lives. They either hold on to their adult children planning for the visits home from college and try to desperately stay active in their children's lives or they realize they have not grown themselves and it is their time to do something with the rest of their life.

Others look at the man they married and realize they have built their lives around their family and responsibilities and have not built a relationship with their husband. These couples should invest their time together now, getting to know each other. Career women have worked and managed a family for many years. One day they realize they have shared their lives together but they don't know each other. Their lives have gone in different directions. It is time to travel and date each other and fall in love again.

As we were preparing to complete our home schooling junior year, our church called and offered me a job. A job! I had not worked in many years as a paid employee. I organized and ran support groups for single parents and for people going through divorce, using my lay counselor skills. But now the church wanted me to take this and other programs further, as an employee. Our family had always been active volunteers at church. The gifts and talents that God gave me to use in his service are organization and creativity. My husband and I both taught Singles Sunday school classes plus our whole family was involved in different aspects of drama productions and coordination of major events. So, I said yes to the job. I began a new adventure with my life as our son went to college. God used this job to teach and develop my computer skills and to expand my event planning into other areas. It was great! However, after several years God decided to push me out of the nest of the church. He had yet another plan for me.

Let me encourage you; always look to the Lord for guidance. Search your heart and seek God in prayer for His desire. Be open to whatever He has for you to do. Don't let fear or finances hold you back. God will provide. Do something using the gifts and talents God gave you. If you don't know what these are, contact my office or go to our web site where you can obtain our test to determine your personality profile, which includes your gifts and talents.

Its time to live, we are in a new season of life. It's a time of celebration!

Natural Therapies

Herbal Formulas and Tips

Vitamin E: 800-1000 IU per day until symptoms have improved, then 400 IU per day. The only clinical studies done on vitamin E were in late 1940s. They found vitamin E to be effective in relieving hot flashes and menopausal vaginal complaints.

Vitamin C: 1200 mg. per day (powder form is best)

Diet: increase the amount of phytoestrogens in the diet by consuming more soy foods, fennel, celery, parsley, flaxseed oil, nuts, and seeds.

Exercise: Regularly, at least 30 minutes three times a week OR jump on a mini trampoline "Trampoline" for 10 minutes which equals a 1 hr. aerobic workout and it is fun.

Hesperidin is flavonoids that are known to improve vascular integrity and relieve capillary permeability. When combined with vitamin C, hesperidin and other citrus flavonoids help in relieving hot flashes. In one clinical study, women were given 900 mg of hesperidin, 300 mg of hesperidin methyl chalcone, a citrus flavonoid, and 1200 mg of vitamin C daily. After taking this dose for one month, symptoms of hot flashes were relieved in 53 percent of the women. In the most recent study, 300 mg per day was the most effective dose to take.Suggested dose is 900 mg per day of Hesperidin with 1200 mg of vitamin C per day.

Gamma-oryzanol (ferulic acid) is a found in grains and rice. It enhances pituitary function and promotes endorphin release by the hypothalamus. 30 mg. per day. In the most recent study 300 mg. per day for 38 days proved to relieve menopause symptoms. Gamma-oryzanol is an extremely safe natural substance with no side effects. It is also effective in lowering blood cholesterol triglyceride levels. Suggested dose is 30 mg. per day.

The most important dietary recommendation is to increase the amount of plant foods, especially those high in phytoestrogens, while reducing the amount of animal foods. Phytoestrogens are plan compounds that are capable of binding to estrogen receptors. Foods high in phytoestrogens include soy, flaxseed, and flaxseed oil, nuts, whole grains, apples, fennel, celery, parsley, and alfalfa. Other cultures that have a diet predominantly plant-based rarely have menopause symptoms. Increasing the intake of dietary phytoestrogens helps decrease hot flashes, increase maturation of vaginal cells and inhibit osteoporosis. One dietary recommendation for relief of hot flashes and atrophic vaginitis is to increase the consumption of soy foods. One cup of soybeans would be equivalent to 0.45 mg or one tablet of Premarin. In my practice it is not uncommon to see clients that added soy to their diets and discovered they were allergic to it. Make sure you are not allergic to soy. Women who consumed the soy foods demonstrated an increase in the number of superficial cells that line the vagina. This increase offsets the vaginal drying and irritation that is common in postmenopausal women.

Exercise regularly, at least 30 minutes three times a week to help reduce the frequency and severity of hot flashes. Ugh! I hate exercise. The theory is endorphin activity within the hypothalamus is a major factor in provoking hot flashes. The study demonstrated that regular physical exercise decreased the frequency and severity of hot flashes. Women who exercised 3.5 hours per week had no hot flash symptoms, but the women who exercised less than that amount had symptoms. Well, since I hate to exercise, I use a Chi machine.

The concept is it brings oxygen and circulation to your body as it moves you from the ankles up in a fish like motion. Yes, I know it sounds too good to be true that 30 minutes on the Chi machine is worth one hour of aerobic exercise. All you do is lay on the floor and the machine does the rest. I also recommend a mini trampoline. Best is a percussion mini trampoline so that when you move slightly up and down, your body does not receive forced impact. 15 minutes on this is worth one hour of aerobic exercise.

Herbal Treatment with Dong Quai, Licorice, Chaste berry, Black Cohosh, and Ginkgo Biloba are proven effective in relieving menopausal symptoms. Dong Quai - 3 times per day. Powdered root or as tea: 1-2 Tincture (1:5): 1 tsp. Fluid extract: 1/4 tsp.

This mixture is used to treat menopausal symptoms, especially hot flashes, painful menstruation, lack of menstruation, too frequent menstruation, and to assure a healthy pregnancy and easy delivery. It causes an increase in uterine contraction, followed by relaxation. Its effectiveness for hot flashes is a combination of Dong Quai's mild estrogenic effects with other components that act to stabilize blood vessels.

Licorice - 3 times per day
Powdered root or as tea: 1-2 g
Fluid extract (1:1) 1 tsp.
Solid extract: 250-400 mg

Licorice is believed to lower estrogen levels while simultaneously raising progesterone levels. For menopause, this estrogen-like activity is responsible for its effects.

Chaste berry - 3 times per day
Powdered berries or as tea: 1-2 g
Fluid extract (1:1) 1 tsp.
Solid extract: 250-500 mg

Caste berry has effects on pituitary function. It also alters LH and FSH secretion during menopause.

Black cohosh - three times per day
Powdered rhizome: 1-2 gm
Tincture (1:5): 4-6 ml
Fluid extract (1:1) 1 tsp. This is based on 2 mg of 27-deoxyactein 2 x's a day
Solid extract: 250-500 mg
The dosage is based on its content of 27-deoxyactein, which serves as an important biochemical marker to indicate therapeutic effect.

A special extract of Cimicifuga racemosa, standardized to contain 1 mg of triterpenes calculated as 27-deoxyactein per tablet (trade name: Remifemin), is the most widely used and thoroughly studied natural alternative to hormone replacement therapy in menopause.

Clinical studies have shown that his Cimicifuga extract relieves not only hot flashes, but also depression and vaginal atrophy.

Ginkgo Biloba - 3 times per day
24% ginkgo flavor glycoside content: 40 mg

Ginkgo Biloba is effective for cold hands and feet, forgetfulness and on the vascular systems. It improves blood flow to the brain, but also enhances energy production in the brain and the transmission of nerve signals. Must take consistently for 12 weeks to see effectiveness.

There are many other natural remedies for menopause and for many other problems that come with menopause. Here are some alternative diagnostic techniques.

Oriental Diagnosis

Oriental methods of diagnosis concentrate mainly on personal touch and observation and very little on outside tests. Some are:

* Pulse-taking
* Tongue diagnosis
* Urine analysis

Western Diagnosis

Western diagnosis uses a combination of both ancient skills and modern "high-tech" machinery and tests. Some of these are:

* Aura reading

* Applied kinesiology

* Iridology

* Reflexology

* Hair analysis

I guess I lean more toward western oriental. I have taken a course on tongue reading, which I found interesting and have used some. I am familiar with pulse-taking. It is a part of Kiki, which is a touch method of balancing your system. I used applied kinesiology before I advanced to computerized testing. I really enjoyed the practice of iridology. I had a special digital iridology camera that would store pictures of the eye for me to analyze later.

Aromatherapy Hot Flash Reducer - As mentioned previously, Clary sage essential oil, used in a diffuser will help to ease hot flashes. Try carrying a handkerchief scented with a drop of clary sage and sniff when symptoms begin. Keep the hankie in a plastic bag so the smell doesn't dissipate. Another tip is to take a lemongrass bath. It is emotionally calming. In addition, before intercourse, you can use jojoba oil to help with dryness. Rose oil is calming for psychological problems; geranium oil mixed with ylang ylang can improve muscle tone when rubbed into the breast; tea tree oil diluted in a concentration 1-3% essential oil to base of olive oil, can also help with vaginal dryness. You can also add 10 drops of oil to a bath.

Diet and Nutrition

All of these aggravate symptoms

As a nutritionist, there are several self-help tips I give my clients.

Avoid caffeine drinks, like cola, coffee, tea

Eliminate dairy products from your diet - but yogurt is okay.

Limit refined carbohydrates

No sugar and sea salt only

Limit spicy foods

No smoking and drinking alcohol

All of these reduce symptoms

Eat raw fruits and raw vegetables

Eat plenty of green vegetables and salads

Eat plenty of calcium rich foods like spinach, oranges, and apples.

Diet is the single most powerful medical therapy available. A low-fat, high-complex-carbohydrate diet is the keystone for treating a number of degenerative diseases. A healthy diet can actually reverse the damage. Your diet should include fruits, vegetables, whole grains, fiber, and soy. Avoid animal products.

Supplements that help

Take Liquid vitamin especially B-6 or B complex, C, and E

Magnesium

Evening primrose oil

Folic acid

Pancreatic enzymes

Zinc

Iron

Homeopathy

Homeopathy deals with mental and physical state of being. Some recommendations might be:

Lachesis, Sepia, Pulsatilla for mood changes

Belladonna for hot flushes

Graphite's for loss of libido/emotional

Cimicifuga for depression, irritability restless

Caulophyllum for nervous tension, anxiety

Arnica for backache, tiredness, aches

Flower Remedy - The emotional issues surrounding menopause are sometimes as difficult as the physical symptoms. The flower remedy Walnut will help one to cross over the bridge with ease. It will help achieve emotional balance during the transition. Another is Aloe Vera for hot flashes. It is soothing, cooling, and helpful for mental and emotional burnout.

Reflexology - work on diaphragm, reproductive system and pituitary, thyroid and adrenal gland reflexes on your feet.

Massage

A regular body massage can enhance general health and vitality, while specialized methods can coax tension from muscles, ease stiff joints, promote healthy circulation of the blood, and stimulate lymphatic drainage to encourage the elimination of wastes from the body. Massage brings a healthy glow to dull skin and keep the body feeling firm. Massage is effective for almost any condition and is particularly helpful for tension headaches, back pain, hyperactivity, and insomnia. There are several types of massage. Know what to ask for:

Shiatsu = pressure-point massage

Therapeutic Massage = soothing strokes and rubbing

Reflexology = for hands and feet

Sports Massage = deep tissue massage

Baby Massage = gentle strokes

MLD = manual lymph drainage is a gentle strokes working specifically on the lymph's

Getting In Shape Nutritionally

Your Bodies Needs

In the beginning, God created heaven, earth, garden, man, and woman. The couple did not have a life of idleness. The ground in the garden was fertile without any chemicals. The garden had a river for pure spring water, trees and plants that bear fruit, seeds, and oxygen. Then, a forbidden fruit tree was spotted. The women saw the fruit. It looked good! It couldn't be all bad for you, so she ate. It's a matter of self-discipline.

Why do you eat what you eat?

Do you eat to satisfy your emotions?

Do you eat for physical comfort?

Does food make you feel good?

Do you eat to satisfy an emotional hunger?

We use food to satisfy a need, to comfort ourselves and others, to socialize, but none of these seem to be for health reasons. Clients would say, if it tastes good, it's not good for you. My husband is a foodie. He loves to cook and eat. The plate he prepares is a beautiful presentation. He eats slowly and enjoys every bite. He is also a heart patient that has no self disciple when it comes to food. I, however, eat because it is a physical requirement for the body.

Think of your body as a car engine. It needs certain things to run!

Water (Use Spring Water)

Gas (Fruit and Vegetable)

Oil (Minerals)

Spark Plugs (Enzymes)

Maintenance (Vitamins)

Understanding the body and its imbalances and disharmonies needs a holistic approach. The word holistic means whole. Each part of the body must interact and work together. The mind can trick the body into believing illness exist and the bodies' nutritional deficiencies can cause emotional upheavals in the mind. Lets look at the basic. What do we need to be in shape nutritionally.

Water
There are many types of water, tap water, well water, spring water,

mineral water, filtered water, and distilled water.

Tap Water: There are 3 advantages of using tap water. 1) convenience 2)available 3)it costs only pennies, but; tap water has many health disadvantages. The water is process in a treatment plant in settling tanks, which filters through sand and gravel. This does not completely make the water pure for drinking. The chemicals used for purification may not clear all the environmental pollutants that contaminate our water. If you must drink tap water, use a filter. Most modern refrigerators have filtration systems.

Spring Water: Drink 64 ounces of spring water a day to replenished the two quarts of water our bodies use. Water is used to maintain our bodily fluids components made up of : blood, lymph, digestive juice, urine, tears and sweat. Water is used for our bodily functions: circulation, digestion, absorption, and elimination. It is very importantly to note that water carries the electrolytes and mineral salts conveying electrical currents in the body. The mineral salts are: sodium, potassium, calcium, magnesium, and chloride.

Distilled Water: There are two schools of though concerning drinking distilled water. Some natural health practitioners feel it is the best and the cleanest water to drink because the distillation process removes all the minerals, organisms, and chemicals from the water, making it pure H20. Other practitioners feel the human body does not use these inorganic minerals. The majority feel by drinking distilled water you can become deficient in minerals. Many minerals that can be used in the body are in the inorganic or salt state and are not part of the organic tissue.

The best drinking water, according to my research, is Reverse Osmosis or Ozonated, which has a high oxygen level. Ozone therapy is a form of alternative medicine treatment that purports to increase the amount of oxygen in the body through the introduction of ozone.

The best way to drink water is in intervals throughout the day. Do not drink a 16 ounce full glass of water before or just after meals. This will dilute digestive juices and reduce food nutrient assimilation.

Water intervals:

      10:00 A.M. -2 cups/16 ounces

      1:00 P.M. - 2 cups/16 ounces

      3:00 P.M. - 2 cups/16 ounces

      5:00 P.M. - 2 cups/16 ounces

Don't drink more than a gallon of water a day, because it becomes a negative and will wash all the minerals out of your system. But if you are dehydrated from lack of water or drinking caffeine, then you need to replace what you have lost. If you drink any alcohol for every 8 ounces, you need to replenish your water level with 16 ounces of water. Alcohol is dehydrating and acidic. Flying on an airplane is very dehydrating. Drink bottled water before, during, and after the flight. It is a plus and minus system. For any minus beverage you drink you must add back in 16 ounces of water to equalize the fluids.

Carbohydrates

A balanced diet includes Carbohydrates. They are a main source of energy. They easily convert to glucose (fuel for our cells). As they role play with the nervous system, muscles and organs. They also regulate protein and fat. In conjunction with protein and fat, they help fight infection, tissue growth and lubricate joints. They are high in fiber, which is beneficial unless you are trying to loose weight or have candida!

The three principals in carbohydrates are:

(1) Sugar: (1) Glucose, which is found in fruits, cane sugar, milk sugar and malt syrup. (2) Fructose, which are fruits, fruit juice, honey, and some vegetables? (3) Lactose, which is milk sugar.

(2) Starches: potatoes, vegetable roots, whole grains such as wheat, rice, and corn.

(3) Fiber: skins of fruits, vegetables, covering on cereals grains (wheat bran), pectin in rind of citrus fruits, pulp of apples.

How are Carbohydrates digested?

Carbohydrates are broken down in the gastrointestinal track by enzymes for absorption into the blood. The lactose, sucrose, and maltose are converted into glucose, fructose, and galactose. Starches are converted by salivary amylase in the mouth into dextrin. The dextrine is reduced to maltose by pancreatic amylase which are released into the small intestine. The small intestinal lining, the maltose, is broken down into glucose by maltase enzymes. The small intestine sucrose is changed into glucose by the enzyme sucrose. The simple sugars, glucose, galactose, and fructose are the product of carbohydrate digestion and are absorbed into the bloodstream through the intestinal lining. The blood then circulates to the liver, where fructose and galactose are converted into floccose and regulated by the liver for use by the cells to make the fuel for energy.

Proteins

Proteins are needed as a component of our muscles, hair, skin, eyes, internal organs, heart muscle and brain. Our immune system needs protein to form antibodies (fighters). We need protein to regulate metabolism (thyroid, insulin) and for body tissue.

Vegetarians or people eliminating protein from their diet for detoxification purposes will not find it difficult to get enough protein particularly if they eat eggs and dairy foods. Without eggs and dairy, a balanced combination of vegetables, grains, nuts, and legumes is needed. Examples are: millet, aduki beans, brown rice, sunflower seeds, soybeans, rice or soybeans with sesame, corn, wheat, rye, peanuts, coconut, legumes or leafy greens with grains. The most important fact is not the protein content but the biological value and how the body utilized the protein in the food.

What are protein builders?

Amino acids-build protein to create body tissue, red blood cells and skin cells. They last one month in the intestinal cells then need to be replaced two times every 6 weeks.

Symptoms of protein deficiency

Weight loss, fluid retention, weakness, hair loss, and inability to heal wounds.

Fats and Oils

Fats and oils are needed for their nutrients. They are found in meats, dairy foods, nuts, seeds, soybeans, olives, peanuts, and avocados.

Functions

Fats and oils are energy reserves which can be burned to make energy when we need it or are not getting enough from our diet. They transport nutrients (Vitamins A, D, E and K). They are a component of the cell membrane and internal fatty tissues that protect the vital organs from trauma by regulating body temperature and insulation. Because of their insolubility in water, fats and oils require our bodies to take special care to digest and transport nutrients to the cells and organs, so as to insulate organs and regulate body temperatures. The chewing process is the first act of digestion to separate fats.

Immune System

The Liver helps protect the body by removing toxic substances from the bloodstream. It activates the enzymes that metabolize the nutrients from food. The nutrients are in turn delivered to every cell in the body, including the cells that make up the immune system. The liver manufactures a substance called bile. It uses the bile to flush itself of poisons accumulated from the bloodstream. The process of metabolism depends on how well your liver is doing.

The Gallbladder is an organ that serves as a storage place for bile. The bile flow in the liver can become hindered from diet. Fiber-poor, mineral deficient and refined sugar diets, tends to produce solid particles from bile components (gallstone).

The Colon is five feet of intestinal tubing known as the large intestine. The common American diet creates a buildup of toxic waste substances coating the walls. Foods such as white bread, cakes, cookies, meat, milk, doughnuts and spaghetti are all fiber poor food that make it hard for the colon to do its job. These and other foods leave a coating of slime on the inner walls of the colon like plaster on a wall. This coating gradually increases in thickness

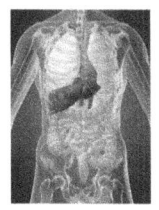 until there is only a small hole through the center. Fiber is our intestinal broom A few symptoms of an unhealthy colon include gas, headaches, irritability, run-down feeling, chronic fatigue, dulled senses, and perceptions. The solution is to cleanse the colon!

Mucus is a normal substance produced in your body to coat the stomach, lubricate the intestines, colon, and aid in elimination. However, the proper foods fruits and vegetables, eaten raw, produce only minimal amounts. Eating foods cooked and processed produce an excessive amount of the mucus. This mucus is sticky. It sticks to the colon walls, building up a layer that become hard and rubber like in consistency. The more harmful foods you eat the more layers you accumulate. These layers prevent the proper exchange of nutrients and toxins, therefore, trapping the toxins where they should not stay and preventing the nutrients and oxygen from getting where they need to go. The proper process is needed for healthy organs and cellular regeneration. Rebuilding and maintaining your body's own natural defense system, depends on rebuilding healthy cells. The key to healthy cells is the unhindered flow of nutrients from the food we eat.

Degenerative diseases are caused by the body's inadequate metabolic response to a condition in which the cells of the body are being slowly poisoned by too many of the wrong things or not enough of the right thing at the right time.

Enzymes

Enzymes supply the energy for all the biochemical reactions upon which life is built, including the digestion of food. Our bodies have digestive enzymes, which are reactivated by the liver! A poor liver equals reduced enzymatic activity, which leads to poor digestion that leads to undernourished cells. Natures plan calls for food enzymes to help with digestion instead of forcing the bodies' own digestive enzymes to carry the whole load.

In raw food, you receive enzymes, vitamins and minerals. In cooked food your body gives up the vitamins, minerals, and enzymes just to get the food processed through your body. The reason we need enzymes is because the biochemical reaction in the body will not function without them. Every organ in our bodies, all the tissues and cells, run on a metabolic process. The driver of this metabolic process is a metabolic enzyme. In order for you to be able to handle the cooked food you eat, your body needs enzymes to process them. If you do not have sufficient enzymes available, your body cannot process properly what you ingest. It will end up in your bloodstream, creating havoc in your body.

TROUBLE IN PARADISE - *Pollutants in Your Body*

In order to get your body totally clean, you must cleanse right down to the cellular level. Cells are the basic building blocks for the body.

They are designed to regenerate themselves, as well as burn fuel and give us energy. This metabolism process also produces a residual waste, which must be carried through our bloodstream to our colon and eliminated. When the system gets all plugged up, it is the start of things that are about to go wrong. There are four steps which every cell in the body should experience daily. Nutrition, oxygen, waste elimination, and renewal. If cells do not get what they need, proper nutrients they cannot regenerate. We are oxygen-burning machines. If a cell does not receive enough oxygen, the cell dies and become another toxin which must be removed from our tissues. If we don't properly eliminate the waste from our cells they become polluted and incubators for disease. When waste products from the blood can't penetrate colon walls, they are re-absorbed into the body that equals autointoxication. The body is poisoning itself. Compound this situation with other toxins. Illness is just a symptom; it is not the disease. The true disease is toxemia, or to put it simply, a toxin-permeated, unclean body, which in it weakened state is unable to defend itself against certain physical attacks. Diseases are symptoms of the root cause, toxemia.

You are probably saying, I don't have time to do all this. Do you eat the five servings of fruit and vegetables daily? Do you eat on the run? Do you skip meals? Are you trying to watch your caloric intake to lose weight? Do you eat out often? Do you need more energy? A solution might be a Green Miracle drink. It is a convenient way to receive the nutrients you may be lacking in your diet. One serving (small scoop) provides over 7,800 mg of nutrients: It has a blend of 40 super foods, an appetite suppressant to curb craving, and it provides increased energy and stamina while building the immune system.

Ionic Trace Minerals

The fluids in our body are almost identical to seawater. Ionic Trace Minerals provides minerals that are 26 times more concentrated and provide over 50 minerals. With the absence of minerals, vitamins cannot function. If we are lacking in vitamins, our system can make use of the minerals, but if lacking in minerals, the vitamins are useless."

The human body can manufacture some vitamins, (B in the intestinal tract, D from sunshine) but the body cannot manufacture its own minerals, they must be supplied by food and water. When minerals are adequate, they make a strong, healthy body. When minerals are lacking, disease sets in. Vitamin and Mineral supplements are to rebuild healthy cells, change body chemistry and reinforce the body's own protective systems. Vitamin and Minerals help restore and reinforce the body's own ability to fight off disease. They are at the deepest levels of the body process, and regenerative changes in body chemistry usually require time to rebuild.

Calling in dietary reinforcements such as supplements is an effort to help supply the body with the right things that it is lacking in order to provide optimum health. It is up to the body to take these nutrients and build healthy cells.It is not enough to feed the body; we must pay attention to the interaction of the parts. We know that electrical frequencies are the driving energizing force in every cell.

Each cell acts as a battery. Each cell has a different electrical charge on the inside. When a nerve cell is stimulated, a wave of depolarization travels down the nerve fiber. Potassium is released and sodium moves into the cell. When that current passes, the cell wall must re-establish the charge difference. A pump gets the potassium back inside the cell again. This battery sets up its own electromagnetic current. The collection of all these electrical forces, about the trillions of our cells, constitutes our energy system. Fatigue may be, your batteries have run down. The cells need glucose and minerals for voltage potential in each cell. The body is a bioelectrical organism. *All the vitamins in the world are worthless unless our body is minerals and bioelectrical balanced.*

The consumption of even small amounts of caffeinated beverages like coffee, tea, and soft drinks increases a person's risk for calcium and magnesium deficiencies.

Sodium is the primary mineral ion found in extra cellular fluids and is essential for the transmission of electrical nerve impulses.

Magnesium is one of the most important components in every cell of the body. Magnesium is required for proper nerve function and the activation of most of the B Vitamin Complex. It is an essential part of many enzyme systems, including the production and transfer of energy for protein synthesis.

MEN

What You Needs to Know about Your Man

What about men, do they really go through a menopause or a mid-life crisis? I call it man-o-pause! Yes, men go through menopause also.

At about age 50 men begin to look at things differently; they get spare tires around their middle. They join a health club, vowing to attend every day and get their body in shape. Their thinking begins to change, they think more about their appearance, the way they dress and look. This is labeled as a mid-life crisis. They may adopt a hairstyle to comb all the hair forward to cover the bald spots that are developing. Others may try to cover the gray, smooth the wrinkles and stay young. Some decide to stay away from middle-aged people, thus leaving their wife for younger women to prove that they are still handsome and attractive. Single men date and want to be seen with younger women.

For many men the responsibilities forced upon them during these years increase they're feeling of losing their youth. I am told this is when some men turn to younger women because it makes them feel youthful, desirable, and more sexually capable of being able to satisfy a young woman. For Christian men, this is a time to rely on the Lord for strength. To keep a focus and to have accountability partners. Help them find a men's groups or Sunday school class where they can become active.

Lucille Morrison from the American Institute of Family Relations, said this to men; "In the twenties we acquire a family; in our thirties we acquire things; in our forties we acquire anxieties."

Men's mid-life crisis does not spring up from a single cause. It represents a cluster of physical, psychological and spiritual symptoms that occur in most men sometime between forty and fifty. Just as women, each man handles it in a different way. In a way, they cross a similar bridge as we do but their bridge is different. They begin to have physical problems. Sexually, men may develop erectile dysfunction and panic sets in. Testosterone, a hormone that makes men virile and sexually alive, begins during puberty. It increases until a man is in his twenties, and after that, decreases very slowly. They do not have a significant change in hormone supply. Usually, sexual problems lie not in the glands but in the head.

Dr. Robert Rose and his associates at the Boston University School of Medicine discovered that the testosterone level of males under stress becomes significantly lower than for those who are not. Stress seems to have a "see-saw relationship", Rose concluded. "As the stress goes up, the testosterone goes down".

Psychologically, by the time men reach there 40's they begin to analyze their life and look at where they have been and where they are going. This is a time when several things happen to them emotionally. They virtually feel trapped between their past and present.

A man may feel they should have been more successful and if they are still trying to accomplish goals, this is the time they sometimes give up and digress emotionally, spiritually, financially, and physically. A man may get passive and feel stuck, not moving in any direction. Alternatively, they just settle for where they are. Usually depression begins. A man may try to recapture their youth and plunge into a new life or new career. He may pick himself up, make changes, and still work at achieving his goals. We, as women, should recognize these things and most of all support the men in our lives. These men could be our husbands, our fathers, close friends, anyone. We need to give them support, attention, love, understanding, no matter how crazy they act. If we have built a relationship of communication over the years, we should be able to help them.

Jesus also commanded that we love our neighbor as ourselves. This is a lot of responsibility for men and women on the bridge. He is saying we need intimacy with others. True intimacy develops out of openness and communication.

People, working through the mid-life, sometimes drop out when they should be cultivating relationships. We need people to care about not merely care for and who care about us. The family is pictured that the man is responsible to care for his wife, his children, and aging parents and to be a rock, with nothing in return. I feel we need to go back to basics and the wife should care and love her husband as she loves Christ. The priority for women should be: Christ, Husband, Children, Self, Family, Church. Scripture tells us we are helpmates, to be along side our husbands

Psychiatrist Paul Meier said, "Every man needs one intimate friend of the opposite sex, preferably his wife, and two friends of the same sex with whom he can share his feelings". Men may need to take a lead from their wives. Overall, women seem better able to establish sharing friendships than men do.

Dr. Meyer Friedman suggests that men make goals at mid-life personal rather than professional. He makes these suggestions.

1. *Things worth being are better than things worth having*
2. *Live by the calendar rather than the stopwatch*
3. *Make each day contain something of memory value*
4. *Each day should have something related to beauty, love, growth, or novelty, this is not a lost day.*

Couples

When a woman has gone through menopause she will notice a glow about her, much like the glow of pregnancy. Her energy is magnetic; she is full of integrity, joy, overflowing with love and has a sense of self-pride and worth. How the man in her life responds to her is an indication of how she will spend the rest of her life. From the time a woman begins premenopausal until post-menopause and then some, she will need one important thing from her man: Support! Loving support when the man in her life has gone off track and she begins to see the signs I have described. Do not confront him or criticize him because that is not what he needs. He needs one thing: your loving support.

The following are some suggestions for couples as to how to spend the rest of your lives together happy, healthy and full of life.

1. Get to know each other without the adult kids or grandkids around.
2. Do not pour yourself into adult children or grandkids, therefore not investing time and interest in each other.
3. Turn off the TV. Sit outside and find something to talk about.
4. Fall in love again, go on dates
5. Send notes to each other
6. Go for a ride on Sunday afternoon
7. Buy flowers, work in your yard together
8. Cook together
9. Encourage each other to develop
10. Don't hold on for fear of loosing them as they grow, let your roles change
11. Don't stay at home, get out and volunteer
12. Start a new project together
13. Let the kids go to start their own life
14. Grow together
15. Travel
16. Buy time shares
17. Find things to do with little money
18. Serve at church as greeters
19. Get active in a class
20. Meet people younger and do things with them
21. Encourage your parents to grow together
22. Let go and start your own life
23. Kids - Encourage your mom to do something with her life

This new energy and clarity partly stems from the absence of premenopausal symptoms. You'll feel better than you have in years. But there's more going on, experts say. Notes OB-GYN Christine Northrup, author of the Wisdom of Menopause: "Our bodies, minds and lives are set up so our best times start after 50." Give yourself permission to explore whom you are and how you want to live during the next chapter of your life. It's time to start putting yourself first.

I hope you have grown in knowledge, become encouraged and have a new focus and direction in life as you travel on the train of life.

Blessing of Health

K. B. LeMere, N.N.D.